Evening Primrose Oil

THE "ESSENTIAL" EFA

Karen Bradstreet

Woodland Publishing
Pleasant Grove, UT

TABLE OF CONTENTS

Evening Primrose Oil

Introduction

The saying, "Good things come in small packages" is especially true when refering to the tiny seeds of the evening primrose flower. These seeds are the source of an oil valued the world over for building health and overcoming many common health problems.

Evening primrose is also known as evening star, night willow herb, scabish, and tree primrose. It boasts a recorded history of at least 500 years of use for its healthful properties. The plant grows in a wide variety of climates, from rocky roadsides, to shallow streams, to high deserts. It will even grow at elevations as high as 9,000 feet. From July to September the plant bears yellow flowers which open after sunset and are pollinated by night-flying insects. The flowers are open only until sunrise the next day and then die—hence the name "evening" primrose.

Once the flower dies, the ovary swells, turns green and hardens. Hundreds of small black seeds form inside. These are the source of the plant's famous oil. About 5,000 seeds are needed to yield enough oil for one 500 mg capsule. For this reason, evening primrose oil is relatively costly.

HISTORY OF EVENING PRIMROSE OIL

American Indians and European immigrants recognized evening primrose's value in a wide variety of ailments. Indians used it to treat skin wounds, asthma, coughs, and as a sedative. It was one of the first botanicals exported to Europe from North America. In 1619, it was brought to Italy and planted in the Padua Botanical Gardens. The Puritans so valued it they dubbed it the "King's cure-all," and exported it to England.

The ancients may not have known scientifically why evening primrose is so effective for so many illnesses, but that didn't make it any less effective. Modern science is providing ever-expanding validation of its beneficial nutritional properties.

The Secret is in the Seeds

The essential fatty acids found in the oil of the evening primrose seeds are the secret to the oil's health-building properties. In order to understand why these essential fatty acids are so important, we first need to understand the body's need for certain types of dietary fats, and the damaging effects the wrong types of dietary fats can have.

Healthy vs. Unhealthy Fats

The "Good" Fats—Essential Fatty Acids

In the past few years, fat has acquired a bad name. But the truth is, while some types of fats are unhealthy, certain types of fat are actually vital for good health. One group of these healthy fats is the essential fatty acids (EFAs). They are found in certain unprocessed vegetable and plant oils, as well as fish oils. A mother's milk is also one of the richest sources known.

Essential fatty acids are nutritional substances, like vitamins and minerals, that have far-reaching effects on many body processes, including the following:

• *Reducing blood pressure*
• *Helping prevent arthritis*
• *Reducing the growth rate of breast cancer*
• *Lowering cholesterol and triglyceride levels*
• *Maintaining healthy skin*
• *Aiding in transmission of nerve impulses*
• *Playing a role in normal brain function*
• *Constituting the building blocks of body membranes*
• *Promoting proper hormone function*
• *Forming the basis for prostaglandin production*

EFAs can't be manufactured by the body and therefore must be consumed in the diet. In a report titled "Dietary Fats and Oils in Human Nutrition," the Food and Agricultural Organization and the World Health Organization recommend that at least three percent of an adult's daily caloric intake be comprised of essential fatty acids. The diets of children and pregnant women should be at least five percent EFAs.

EFAs are essential to the normal functioning of all body tissues. In fact, because of their many functions, the list of symptoms of essential fatty acid deficiency is a long one. It includes, but is not limited to:

• *reduced growth rate*
• *skin disorders—dryness, eczema, scaliness, flakiness*
• *male and female infertility*
• *kidney abnormalities*

- *decreased capillary resistance*
- *susceptibility to infection*
- *heart problems*
- *anemia*
- *enlarged, fatty liver*
- *sparse hair growth in infants*
- *poor wound healing*
- *increased susceptibility to infection*

In order to prevent or to heal these conditions, a diet rich in EFAs must be a priority. There are several types of essential fatty acids. They include:

Linoleic acid: This is found in the seeds of sunflower, safflower, corn, soy and evening primrose.

Gamma-linolenic acid: Rich sources are human milk, evening primrose, and black currant seeds.

Diho-mogamma-linolenic acid: Small amounts are found in human milk and organ meats such as the adrenals, spleen and kidneys.

Arachadonic acid: This EFA is found in meats, dairy products, shrimp, prawns, and some seaweeds.

Alpha-linolenic acid: This is found in green leafy vegetables. Linseed oil contains large amounts and soy contains small amounts.

Elcosapentaeonic acid: This EFA is found mostly in fish oils such as herring and salmon.

The two EFAs that are in the spotlight these days are linoleic acid and gamma-linolenic acid, or GLA. One reason these essential fatty acids are important to health is that they help balance the body's production of important chemical substances called prostaglandins. Linoleic acid is a precursor from which gamma-linolenic acid is formed in the body. Evening primrose oil is a good source of both. The average evening primrose oil on the market today contains about 72 percent linoleic acid and 9 percent gamma-linolenic acid.[1]

Prostaglandin Production and Essential Fatty Acids

Prostaglandins are highly active hormonelike substances formed in the body from unsaturated fatty acids. They're classified somewhat like vitamins. The major prostaglandins have been grouped into four categories, identified as prostaglandins A, B, E and F. They are classed according to their chemical constituents and subdivided according to the number of bonds in their molecule chains. (In this booklet, notations for various prostaglandins follow this pattern: prostaglandin E1 is noted as PGE1, prostaglandin A2 is noted as PGA2, etc.) Scientists know of the existence of about 20 different prostaglandins.

There is still a lot that science doesn't know about prostaglandins, but in the past few years knowledge has steadily increased. Interest first began in 1930 after it was observed that human semen had certain properties that could relax or contract the uterus. It was determined that the prostate gland contains high amounts of these properties, so they were named prostaglandins after the prostate gland. Researchers over the past several decades have delved into understanding the function of prostaglandins. Some recent findings indicate that prostaglandins:

- *influence hormones and affect body processes at the cellular level*
- *can contract or relax smooth muscles of the female reproductive system*
- *may affect relaxation and contraction of the intestinal tract, bronchi, and cardiovascular system*
- *influence gastric secretion and kidney function*
- *affect the health of skin*

Different prostaglandins work in different ways. For instance, PGE1—the prostaglandin most noted for health benefits[2]—does all of the following:

- *lowers blood pressure*
- *opens blood vessels*
- *relieves angina pain*
- *slows cholesterol production*
- *enhances effectiveness of insulin*
- *prevents inflammation*
- *controls arthritis*
- *produces a sense of well-being*
- *stops the growth of some types of cancer cells*

Some scientists believe the therapeutic potential of prostaglandins is even greater than that of steroids. Experimental studies show potential in the following areas[3]:

- *inducing labor at term*
- *preventing premature labor*
- *inducing menstruation*
- *increasing fertility in some circumstances*
- *managing some types of hypertension*

- *controlling some types of cardiac arrythmias*
- *correcting some red blood cell defects*
- *controlling asthmatic seizures*
- *inhibiting gastric secretions in the treatment of gastric ulcers*

Because prostaglandins have so many effects on the body, when we develop either an excess or a deficiency, we become susceptible to a staggering number of health problems. Inflammatory diseases such as arthritis or multiple sclerosis are a common result of a deficiency because prostaglandins help control inflammation in the body. In fact, anti-inflammatory drugs like aspirin work by blocking the body's synthesis of certain prostaglandins.

Science has successfully created synthetic prostaglandins for use as drugs. However, because prostaglandins have such wide-ranging effects, using them involves some risk. For instance, a prostaglandin taken to induce labor may have undesirable effects on other body processes.

Taking a natural nutritional substance that helps the body produce prostaglandins is a much safer alternative. This is where evening primrose comes in. Evening primose oil provides the raw materials—the essential fatty acids—which the body needs to manufacture important prostaglandins.

"BAD" FATS—SATURATED FATS, HYDROGENATED OILS AND TRANS-FATTY ACIDS

The terms "saturated" and "unsaturated" fats have become household words, but do we really know what they mean? In simple terms, *saturated* fats have all the hydrogen atoms they can handle. This full load of hydrogen makes them solid at room temperature. All animal fats are saturated, as are the oils of palm and coconut. Saturated fat is a well-known culprit of heart disease. As a result, just about everyone has heard the dietary recommendation to eat less red meat because it is high in saturated fat. Movie popcorn has also been attacked because it's popped with coconut oil, a highly saturated fat.

Unsaturated fats, on the other hand, do not have all the hydrogen atoms they can handle and are liquid at room temperature. Unsaturated fats come mostly from vegetables and fish. Depending on how many hydrogen atoms they lack, they're classified as polyunsaturated (corn, safflower, and sesame oil) or monounsaturated (olive oil). Essential fatty acids are polyunsaturated. Both polyunsaturated and monounsaturated fats become rancid more quickly than saturated fats because in the absence of hydrogen, their carbon atoms react more readily with oxygen.

Hydrogenation, the widespread process of forcibly adding hydrogen atoms to unsaturated fats and oils, was developed to lengthen shelf life and create the solid fats people like to cook with. Margarines and shortenings are often hydrogenated to give them a longer shelf-life and increase cooking appeal. If you are a label reader, you will notice the word "hydrogenated" on most oils you buy, even cooking oils.

Hydrogenation, like other modern food processing techniques, seems like a great idea. It can prevent spoilage for years! However, in recent years hydrogenation has become a health issue because studies show hydrogenated oils are harmful to health. One reason is that they undergo chemical changes during processing that make them foreign to the body's normal biologic processes. The body simply doesn't know what to do with them, so they create unhealthy cellular activity. They have even been described as acting like plastic in the body.

Specifically, hydrogenation creates substances called trans-fatty acids, which are currently making the front-page news as a prime suspect in heart disease. Most notably for our discussion, they make it hard for the body to convert linoleic acid to linolenic acid.

ANTAGONISTS IN PROSTAGLANDIN PRODUCTION

With the abundance of food available today in Western nations, is anyone really at risk for being deficient in essential fatty acids? And is prostaglandin malfunction really a problem? The answer to both questions is definitely "yes." Although we have an abundance of food, many of the foods we eat—in particular, processed fats and oils like those found in french fries and packaged cookies—are antagonistic to essential fatty acid metabolism in the body, and therefore to prostaglandin production.

Almost all processed foods that contain fat contain these unhealthy hydrogenated oils. In addition, most vegetable oils purchased for cooking are hydrogenated. The following list of food items, which all contain hydrogenated oils, shows just how widespread these oils are:

- *packaged potato mixes*
- *stuffing/breading mixes*
- *bottled and canned gravies*
- *crackers*
- *granola cereals*
- *flavored instant coffee mixes*
- *packaged rice mixes*
- *frozen vegetables in sauce*
- *refried beans*
- *microwave popcorn*
- *non-dairy creamers*
- *toaster pastries*

As you can see, the consumption of unhealthy oils is incredibly widespread. In fact, chances are that most people in industrialized societies eat almost solely unhealthy oils. We eat very few healthy oils at all, such as olive oil or unprocessed, unhydrogenated plant oils. That's why so many people are at risk for health problems linked to EFA deficiency.

Eating too many unhealthy fats isn't the only cause of inadequate GLA production. Other causes include moderate to high alcohol consumption; natural loss of ability to manufacture GLA due to aging; lack of dietary zinc, magnesium and vitamin B6, which are necessary for GLA formation; viral infections; radiation; and cancer. Increasing the dietary intake of EFAs can help overcome these problems.

Therapeutic Applications of Evening Primrose Oil

Including essential fatty acids in the diet (evening primrose oil being an important source) can have powerful health benefits. From the late 1970s to the early 1990s, more than 250 scientific papers were written about the health benefits of evening primrose oil. This oil can help improve various health conditions, some of which are listed below in alphabetical order.

For optimal health, use evening primrose oil as part of a diet which limits the intake of processed oils, white flour products, and sugar, but increases the number and variety of fresh fruits, vegetables, and grains. Keep in mind that many, if not most, health problems are linked to overconsumption of unhealthy foods and underconsumption of healthy ones. These same dietary suggestions would apply to the following health conditions.

For most conditions, expect to take evening primrose oil for six to eight weeks before you see a significant improvement in health. The standard therapeutic dose is four grams per day (four to eight capsules).

ACNE

Acne affects eighty percent of people between twelve and twenty-four. Women are sometimes plagued with it into their thirties and beyond. It occurs when the sebaceous glands, located in each hair follicle, become clogged with the oil that normally lubricates the skin. The trapped oil becomes a prime place for bacteria to multiply, resulting in inflammation. It is common in adolescence because of hormones that stimulate oil production.

Although acne is considered a rite of passage for adolescents in "developed" nations, it is rare in some countries. The Canadian Eskimos, for instance, didn't develop acne until recent decades when their diets began to include standard junk food— sugar and refined carbohydrates. Those foods are usually part of an ingredient panel that includes refined oil which, as mentioned earlier, is antagonistic to essential fatty acids and overall nutrition.

Evening primrose oil has shown promise in treating acne by supplying the gamma-linolenic acids the skin needs for good health and repair.[4] Results are especially promising when it is combined with supplemental zinc.

ALCOHOLISM

Alcohol is a poison that damages the brain, liver, pancreas, duodenum, and central nervous system. It is well-known today that alcohol is toxic to the developing fetus and should be avoided altogether by pregnant women.

Because alcohol blocks the conversion of linoleic acid to gamma-linolenic acid, it can create a GLA deficiency in the body. Some suggest that alcoholics drink to maintain healthy levels of PGE1 levels in the brain, because PGE1 affects moods. It is theorized that raising the alcoholic's levels of PGE1 may decrease the craving for alcohol. Evening primrose oil has also been studied for reducing the symptoms of alcohol withdrawal, preventing liver damage and preventing central nervous system impairment.[5]

The results are promising. In a double-blind study at Craig Dunain Hospital, a group of alcoholics who were given evening primrose oil while going through withdrawal reported less intense withdrawal symptoms.[6] The recommended dosage is 1/2 to 1 gram three times daily.

AUTOIMMUNE DISORDERS

Autoimmune diseases, such as multiple sclerosis, rheumatoid arthritis, asthma, migraines, and ulcerative colitis, can be greatly influenced by evening primrose oil. This oil contains prostaglandins which affect a large variety of the body's immune and inflammatory responses.

Prostaglandin action affects the immune system's T-cell activity. T-cells are cells which appear to ensure that our immune system attacks only foreign invaders, and not the body's own cells. When something goes wrong with this system, the body may begin attacking its own cells. This is believed to be a root cause behind autoimmune diseases. Those suffering from these diseases also show an increased level PGE 2.

Those who suffer from inflammatory diseases often take aspirin to relieve pain and inflammation. Ironically, aspirin actually creates a further prostaglandin imbalance. A more sound approach is to balance the body's prostaglandin production nutritionally, using evening primrose oil. Several studies cited under various disease headings in this booklet document evening primrose oil's value in treating inflammatory diseases.

BRITTLE FINGERNAILS

Findings published in the May 1981 *British Journal of Dermatology* suggest that evening primrose oil offers remarkable benefits for those who suffer from brittle fingernails. In fact, the benefits are so consistent that it is now thought that brittle nails may be a sign of essential fatty acid deficiency. In the aforementioned study, brittle fingernails became harder and more normal within two to six weeks after dietary supplementation with evening primrose oil.[7]

CANCER

There is a strong link between high-fat diets and cancer—not just any fat, of course, but the processed fats discussed earlier. Such fats interfere with normal prostaglandin metabolism, which is believed to play a role in the development of cancer. Some forms of cancer are linked to the body's inability to manufacture PGE1. Cancer cells lose the ability to make gamma-linolenic acid, and therefore PGE1. When PGE1 is added to damaged cells, they begin to multiply correctly.[8]

By restoring normal prostaglandin function, evening primrose oil may reverse cancerous conditions. In one study, a carcinogen was administered to rats. Some rats also received supplemental gamma-linolenic acid. Bone marrow smears showed significant damage only to the rats not receiving GLA.[9] In another study,

GLA was added in vitro to three different types of malignant cells. The growth rate of the cancers were markedly reduced.[10]

DANDRUFF

Dandruff is a chronic condition in which the scalp and eyebrows are itchy, inflamed, and slough off dry flakes of skin. Essential fatty acid deficiency is one among many possible causes of dandruff, as is overconsumption of processed fats and oils. Evening primrose oil is beneficial for almost all skin conditions marked by dryness, flakiness, and scaling. (See *Eczema, Psoriasis.*)

DEPRESSION

Fatigue, irritability, hostility, crying, loss of interest in life, and persistent sadness are all symptoms of depression. Most people will experience some or all of these symptoms at some time in their life. Researchers believe a deficiency in a prostaglandin known as E1 is linked to depression. Because evening primrose oil's gamma-linolenic acid is a precursor to PGE1, it shows promise for those suffering from depression. Recommended dosage is one gram three times daily.

DIABETES

In the most simple of terms, diabetes is a disease caused by insulin deficiency and characterized by excess sugar in the blood and urine. Symptoms include the need to urinate frequently, excessive thirst, dizziness, and sugar intolerance. It can begin in childhood or strike later in adulthood. Potential complications of diabetes include kidney problems, amputation of limbs because of circulatory problems, and blindness.

Evening primrose oil helps the body manufacture PGE1, which has insulinlike actions. This may explain, in part, why evening primrose oil is of benefit to diabetics.

In one experimental double-blind study, twenty-two diabetics who suffered from neuropathy were given either four grams of evening primrose oil daily, or a placebo. After six months, the group using the oil improved, while the placebo group worsened.[11]

Studies also suggest that, compared to control patients treated with a standard diabetic diet, patients with type II diabetes can prevent retinopathy and macrovascular complication by eating a diet enriched with linoleic acid.[12] In one controlled study, half a group of 102 newly diagnosed diabetics were placed on a standard Western diet, while the others were on a diet fortified with linoleic acid. Those on the linoleic-acid fortified diet suffered a lower incidence of circulatory complications.[13]

DIAPER RASH

Diaper rash affects just about every baby at some time in his or her development. When urine and stools mix and rest against the skin, pH changes irritate the skin and can lead to a rash. About half of all diaper rashes go away on their own within 24 hours, but the other half can last ten days or longer. In addition to the standard treatments of airing out the baby's bottom, exposing the child to sun, and keeping the skin dry, supplemental evening primrose oil may make baby's skin more resistant.

Babies deficient in EFAs, or whose nursing mothers are deficient, may be more susceptible to diaper rash. Breastfed babies are less likely to get diaper rash because breast milk is rich in essential fatty acids; formula-fed babies have less protection.

Nutritional experts recommend one capsule of evening primrose oil twice daily for the baby.[14]

ECZEMA

Eczema is a skin disorder characterized by inflammation, scaliness, and itchiness. It may be linked to the sufferer's reduced ability to convert linoleic acid to gamma linolenic acid. Because evening primrose oil contains gamma linolenic acid, it can produce dramatic results for eczema sufferers.

A study in the 1987 *Journal of Dermatology* found that eczema patients showed significant improvement after they were treated with evening primrose oil, and they were less dependent on steroids.[15] In another study, sixty adults and thirty-nine children received evening primrose oil and a placebo for twelve weeks in random order and at various doses. Itching was significantly decreased with both low and high doses.[16] Two grams of evening primrose are recommended daily.

ENDOMETRIOSIS

Endometriosis is a potentially debilitating disease in which endometrial tissue grows outside the uterus and attaches itself to other organs, such as the fallopian tubes and ovaries. Pain results when the endometrial tissue swells and bleeds in response to hormonal stimulation during menstruation. Endometriosis affects approximately twelve million American women—approximately ten percent of female adults.

One of the key causes of the pain associated with endometriosis is overproduction of prostaglandins. Evening primrose oil provides the raw materials to help the body balance prostaglandin production, thereby offering benefits to the endometriosis sufferer. Women with endometriosis should also strictly adhere to a diet of whole grains and fresh fruits and vegetables, while avoiding animal products.

FIBROCYSTIC BREAST DISEASE

As many as fifty percent of all adult women suffer from fibrocystic breasts at some time during their reproductive years. The disease is characterized by painful, tender lumps (cysts) in the breasts, especially before the menstrual cycle. Unlike cancerous growths, the cysts move freely.

Evening primrose oil is one of the most successful treatments known for this disease. In a study of 291 patients with severe breast pain, forty-five percent experienced improvement after supplementing their diets with evening primrose oil.[17]

In another study, forty-one patients with cyclical breast pain were treated with evening primrose oil. After two months, they noticed significant improvement in breast tenderness, general well-being, irritability and breast nodules. There were no substantial side-effects and the improvement lasted up to eighteen months with continued supplementation.[0]

Women suffering from fibrocystic disease should eliminate all caffeine from their diet and supplement with high levels of evening primrose oil. The recommended amount is two capsules three times daily.

INFERTILITY

Infertility, generally speaking, is a couple's inability to conceive a child after a year of unprotected intercourse. The acceptable timetable varies depending on the couple's health and age. Some types of infertility may be linked to essential fatty acid deficiency and subsequent prostaglandin imbalance. Some experts speculate, for instance, that prostaglandin malfunction may cause the fallopian tubes to spasm, throwing off the progression of the egg.

Another function of prostaglandins is to induce ovulation. The high level of progesterone characteristic of ovulation triggers prostaglandins, and is a sign ovulation has taken place. An imbalance could prevent ovulation.

Knowledge of exactly what role prostaglandins play in fertility is still in the early stages. We do know that animals deprived of essential fatty acids rapidly become infertile. Researchers believe many types of infertility may eventually be treated with prostaglandins. Simply understanding the link between evening primrose oil and healthy prostaglandin function is a compelling reason for infertile couples to supplement their diet with evening primrose oil.

HEART AND CIRCULATORY PROBLEMS

Several studies have convincingly shown that individuals whose diets contain increased levels of linoleic acid and reduced saturated fats have significantly lower cholesterol levels. According to *Modern Nutrition in Health and Disease,* "Some of these effects can be explained by an improvement in prostaglandin synthesis, but many other complicated biochemical pathways are involved but not yet sufficiently understood to justify a definite explanation of the favorable effects of linoleic acid on the prevention of atherosclerosis."[19] A Canadian study found that patients who took four grams of evening primrose oil daily experienced a 31.5 percent decline in cholesterol after three months of treatment.[20]

When GLA production is inhibited in the body by consumption of alcohol, intake of trans-fatty acids, or deficiency of zinc, magnesium or vitamin B6, evening primrose is recognized as a valuable precursor to prostaglandin production and has a preventive effect on hardening of the arteries (atherosclerosis).[21] Evening primrose oil may also prevent pregnancy-induced high blood pressure, according to one study.[22] It also lowers sodium-induced high blood pressure and improves blood platelet function.[23] The standard recommended amount is three or four 500 mg capsules morning and evening.

HYPERACTIVITY

Hyperactive children are like the Energizer bunny—they keep going, and going, and going—much to their parents' despair. Hyperactivity is strongly linked to diet. Refined sugars, flours, and food additives can cause powerful behavioral changes in children. Hyperactive children who are put on a wholesome diet often show dramatic change.

In addition to giving the hyperactive child the most wholesome diet possible (fresh fruits, vegetables, whole grains, raw nuts and seeds), evening primrose oil is a desirable dietary addition. Excellent results have been noted when evening primrose oil is rubbed directly into a child's skin. A hyperactive British boy who had been threatened to be kicked out of school for intolerable behavior began to use evening primrose oil. After he was on the treatment two weeks, his teacher—who didn't know he was taking the evening primrose oil—said she'd never seen such a dramatic change in a child's behavior.[24]

INFLAMMATION

Dr. John Vane of Wellcome Research Labs is credited with the discovery of the link between prostaglandins and inflammation. In 1971, Dr. Vane discovered that aspirin's effectiveness lies in its ability to block the synthesis of two types of prostaglandins. Based on his findings, it was deduced that prostaglandins play a role in fever, inflammation and pain.

Because it provides the raw material for healthy prostaglandin function, evening primrose oil helps reduce inflammation naturally. This natural alternative is preferable to anti-inflammatory drugs because synthetic drugs have side-effects. Aspirin, for instance, can damage the stomach lining and lead to ulceration. Drugs like acetaminophen can cause kidney disease.

Two different studies with rats showed significant decrease in chronic inflammation when their diets were supplemented with evening primrose oil.[25]

MULTIPLE SCLEROSIS

Multiple sclerosis (MS) is a disease of the central nervous system which destroys the myelin sheaths that cover each nerve, creating inflammation. Symptoms include blurred vision, dizziness, numbness, weakness, tremors, slurred speech, and staggering. The underlying cause of the disease is unknown; therefore, there is no known cure. Stress and poor nutrition may contribute to its onset. It usually occurs in individuals between the ages of 25 and 40. A characteristic of the disease is that it can go into remission for periods of time, only to reappear.

Current research is investigating the possibility that multiple sclerosis is at least partially caused by prostaglandin deficiency. Prostaglandins, of course, are created from essential fatty acids.

In one study, sixteen patients suffering from multiple sclerosis were supplemented with four grams of evening primrose oil daily. After three weeks, they showed improvement in grip strength.[26]

British scientist R.H.S. Thompson showed that the brain tissues in blood cells of some MS patients have reduced levels of linoleic acid. This may be one reason that a thirty percent success rate is reported in Europe for use of evening primrose oil for MS. A British group of MS sufferers called Action for Research of Multiple Sclerosis reports gathering evidence that evening primrose oil slows the progression of multiple sclerosis.[27] The generally recommended amount is two capsules three times daily.

OBESITY

Evening primrose oil appears to increase the activity of brown fat in the body and assist with weight loss. At least two studies have borne this out.

In one of the studies, extremely obese patients lost significant amounts of weight after using supplemental evening primrose oil. Tests revealed that brown fat activity increased dramatically after three to four weeks of supplementation. In another study, thirty-two people supplemented their diets with two grams of evening primrose oil daily, while other people took four and eight grams daily. After six to eight weeks, about half of the subjects who were ten percent over their ideal weight lost pounds. Those who took eight grams daily lost more weight than those who took four grams.[28] The recommended daily amount of evening primrose is four to eight grams.

PARKINSON'S DISEASE

Parkinson's disease is a degenerative disease of the nervous system that appears when there is an imbalance in the chemicals dopamine and acetylcholine in the brain. Symptoms include loss of appetite, tremors, impaired speech and a fixed facial expression. A preliminary study suggests that evening primrose oil supplementation may reduce the tremors associated with Parkinson's disease.[29]

PMS

Women who suffer from PMS have been found to be deficient in PGE1, an anti-inflammatory prostaglandin whose production is inhibited by saturated animal fat and trans-fatty acids (see discussion of processed oils). Evening primrose oil enhances the production of PGE1, and is therefore beneficial for easing PMS discomforts for many PMS sufferers.[30]

Several studies have confirmed evening primrose oil's usefulness to PMS sufferers. In one study, thirty patients with severe PMS received 1,500 mg of evening primrose oil or a placebo twice daily. After four menstrual cycles, those taking evening primrose oil showed decreased symptoms compared to the placebo group.[31]

In an experimental double-blind crossover study, patients treated with evening primrose oil saw sixty percent improvement, compared to forty percent with those using a placebo. The greatest improvement was in the symptoms of irritability and depression.[32]

Another study involved sixty-eight patients with severe PMS who didn't improve while using medications or vitamin B6 therapy (a standard treatment). They were given one to two grams of evening primrose oil starting three days before symptoms began and continuing until the onset of menstruation. Sixty-one percent reported full relief of symptoms; twenty-three percent reported partial relief.[33] The recommended amount of evening primrose oil is one gram three times daily.

PROSTATE DISORDERS: BENIGN PROSTATIC HYPERTROPHY AND PROSTATIS

Benign prostatic hypertrophy (BPH) is the technical name for an enlarged prostate gland. Prostatis—an inflamed, swollen prostate—is usually caused by infection. Symptoms of both these conditions include painful and frequent urination, incontinence, inability to fully empty the bladder, impotence, back pain, painful orgasm, and painful bowel elimination.

Two capsules of evening primrose oil three times daily are recommended as part of an overall dietary program. Supplemental zinc is essential to help overcome BPH and prostatis.

PSORIASIS

Psoriasis is a skin disease characterized by patches of scaly skin, most commonly on the knees, elbows and scalp, but possible anywhere on the body. Symptoms often flare up and then go into remission, and arthritis may be present. It is considered essentially incurable by conventional methods, but dietary methods offer considerable hope. Treatment with steroids is common, but steroids offer no real cure.

It is known that an essential fatty acid deficiency in humans results in skin rashes that resemble eczema and psoriasis. Evening primrose oil is among the natural therapeutic agents for psoriasis because of its rich EFA content. Some psoriasis suffer-ers also see improvement by eliminating the harmful dietary fats discussed earlier (fried foods, margarine, hydrogenated oils) because such fats interfere with normal EFA metabolism.

RAYNAUD'S DISEASE

Considered an autoimmune disorder, Raynaud's disease is characterized by poor circulation in the hands and feet, leading to cold and numbness.

Several Raynaud's disease patients showed improvement after six to eight weeks of supplementation with evening primrose oil. In cold weather, those using evening primrose oil experienced less severe attacks and decreased hand coldness. They also felt more energy and decreased depression.[34]

RHEUMATOID ARTHRITIS

A malady that afflicts mostly older people, rheumatoid arthri-tis is characterized by joint inflammation, most notably of the fingers, knees, wrists, elbows, toes, hips and shoulders. Symptoms include pain, swelling and stiffness. More chronic cases may cause deformation of joints. Arthritis may come on gradually or all at once.

Studies using evening primrose oil suggest that it takes four to twelve weeks to see improvement in rheumatoid arthritis patients. In some patients, the progression of the disease may be completely stopped (although some patients may experience a worsening of symptoms the first one or two weeks). Several patients given 2.1 grams of evening primrose oil daily showed improvement after three months of treatment.[35] The recom-mended dosage is one gram four times daily.

SCHIZOPHRENIA

Symptoms of schizophrenia include feeling detached from reality, lowered emotional response, hallucinations and delusions. It affects about three percent of all people at some time in their lives. Some people have no symptoms until they suffer a trauma; some cases progress slowly and steadily.

Schizophrenia occurs because of an imbalance in the biochemistry of nerve impulses. Nutritional imbalance likely plays a key role. Some research suggests faulty essential fatty acid metabolism as a prime suspect. In 1981 a study by Donald O. Rudin from the Department of Molecular Biology at Eastern Pennsylvania Psychiatric Institute showed a positive response in patients given two to six tablespoons per day of linseed oil, which, like evening primrose oil, contains essential fatty acids.[36]

In another study, six patients were treated with evening primrose oil and penicillin, and all drug treatments were stopped. After sixteen weeks, several patients showed impressive improvement.[37] Evening primrose oil is recommended at three to six grams per day.

SCLERODERMA

Scleroderma, a disease found mostly in women, is characterized by shrinking of the skin. It can eventually attack internal organs. In one study, four women who had scleroderma for five to thirteen years received one gram of evening primrose oil three times daily. After a year, they showed relief of pain in the extremities, improved skin texture and healing of ulcers. It is believed six grams daily may offer even better results.[38]

Conclusion

Essential fatty acids are known to play a vital role in overall health. Evening primrose oil is an key source of EFAs. It can play an important part in the healing of various disease and disorders, because it helps the body to maintain a balance of prostaglandins that are necessary for health. Daily doses of evening primrose can only be beneficial.

Endnotes

1. Brigitte Mars, "Evening Primrose Oil: Rich Source of Essential Fatty Acids," Let's Live, May 1995, 24.
2. Alan Donald, "The Powerful Healing Magic of Evening Primrose," reprinted from Best Ways, September, 1981.
3. Varro E. Tyler, Lynn R. Brady, James E. Robbers, Pharmacognosy, Lea & Febiger, 1981.
4. James F. & Phyllis A. Balch, Prescription for Nutritional Healing, Avery Publishing Group, 1990, 66.
5. Melvyn R. Werbach, M.D., Nutritional Influences on Illness: A Sourcebook of Clinical Research, 1988, 18, 19.
6. Bestways, May 1897.
7. Evening Primrose Oil, Keats Publishing, ©1981, 23.
8. Alan Donald, "The Powerful Healing Magic of Evening Primrose," reprinted from Best Ways, September 1981.
9. Nutritional Influences on Illness, 114.
10. Ibid., 114.
11. Ibid., 180.
12. Maurice Shils & Vernon Young, Modern Nutrition in Health and Disease, Lea & Febiger, 1988, 101.
13. Nutritional Influences on Illness, 180.
14. Dr. Ross Trattler, Better Health Through Natural Healing, McGraw Hill, 1985, 217.
15. Earl Mindell, Earl Mindell's Herb Bible, 90.
16. Nutritional Influences on Illness, 186-187.
17. Ibid., 196.
18. Ibid., 196.
19. Modern Nutrition in Health and Disease, 103.
20. Earl Mindell's Herb Bible, 90-91.
21. Nutritional Influences on Illness, 70.
22. Ibid., 363.

23. Ibid., 101.

24. Alan Donald, "The Powerful Healing Magic of Evening Primrose," reprinted from Best Ways, September 1981.

25. Nutritional Influences on Illness, 268.

26. Ibid., 306.

27. "Down the Path to Healing with Evening Primrose Oil," Nutrition News, Vol. V No. 4, 1982.

28. Nutritional Influences on Illness, 320-321.

29. Ibid., 348.

30. Better Health Through Natural Healing, 489-490.

31. Nutritional Influences on Illness, 369.

32. Ibid., 369.

33. Ibid., 369.

34. Ibid., 374.

35. Ibid., 388-389.

36. Better Health Through Natural Healing, 512.

37. Nutritional Influences on Disease, 402.

38. Ibid., 407.